THE **UNVEILED OBESITY** SOLUTION

Break Free from Food Temptations, Shed Pounds and Energize Your Life

By

DR CHAD L. WATSON

DISCLAIMER

Copyright © 2024 by Dr. Chad L. Watson

Legal & Disclaim

The information provided in this book is intended for educational and informational purposes only. It is not intended to replace professional medical advice, diagnosis, or treatment. Always seek the advice of your physician or qualified healthcare provider with any questions you may have regarding a medical condition. The author and publisher of this book do not assume any liability for any potential consequences resulting from the use of the information presented herein.

TABLE OF CONTENTS

Introduction: Navigating the Weight of the Obesity Crisis

In a world where the scale of obesity looms larger than ever before, the gravity of its impact extends far beyond the mere numbers reflected on a weighing scale.

It casts a formidable shadow over the health and well-being of individuals and communities worldwide, presenting multifaceted challenges that demand urgent attention and innovative solutions.

Imagine a landscape where the relentless surge of obesity not only jeopardizes physical health but also undermines mental well-being, strains social dynamics, and burdens economies with soaring healthcare costs.

It's a landscape where individuals, irrespective of gender, race, or socioeconomic status, find themselves ensnared in a complex web of genetic predispositions, environmental influences, and lifestyle choices, leading to a myriad of health complications.

But what are the driving forces behind this epidemic? What are the current theories on the causes of obesity? Is it solely a result of overeating and sedentary lifestyles, or are there deeper underlying factors at play?

Moreover, emerging research suggests that environmental factors, such as exposure to PFAS (per- and polyfluoroalkyl substances), may also contribute to obesity. Can PFAS truly cause obesity, and if so, how?

Furthermore, could a lack of sun exposure be a contributing factor to obesity?

The interplay between sunlight, vitamin D levels, and metabolic processes raises intriguing questions about the potential role of sunlight in obesity prevention and management.

As we navigate through these questions, another arises: Would expanding Medicare coverage to include weight loss drugs be a cost-effective solution for treating obesity?

Can pharmaceutical interventions truly address the complexities of this multifaceted condition?

But the impact of obesity extends beyond physical health. It also affects quality of life, with snoring being one of the common manifestations. Why does obesity cause snoring, and is there a correlation between being fat and snoring?

Exploring these questions sheds light on the intricate relationship between obesity and sleep-related disorders.

Moreover, what makes someone's voice deep and husky? Are there underlying physiological mechanisms that contribute to this condition, aside from obesity or smoking habits?

Amidst these inquiries, individuals may question their own classification – am I obese or overweight? Despite weighing 225 pounds and standing at 5'9", the distinction between overweight and obese may not always be clear-cut.

In the realm of medical classification, what is the highest class of obesity, and how does it impact individuals' health and well-being?

Finally, why is there a stigma around obesity despite it being considered a medical condition?

This societal stigma adds another layer of complexity to the obesity crisis, affecting individuals' self-esteem, social interactions, and access to healthcare.

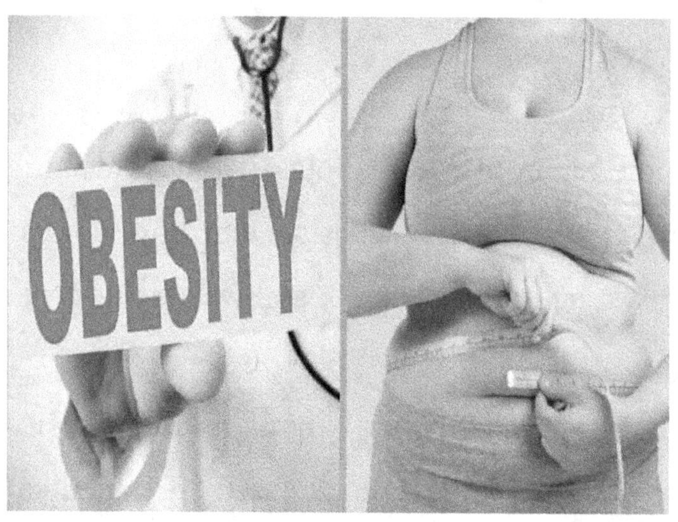

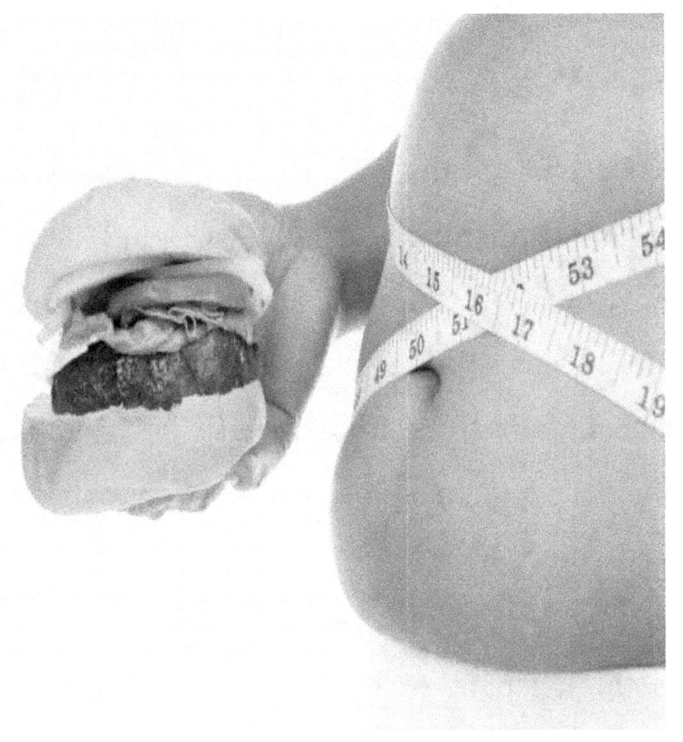

Chapter 1: The Obesity Epidemic Unveiled

Embarking on this journey to understand the obesity epidemic feels like stepping into a labyrinth of tangled truths and hidden consequences. It's a reality that touches every aspect of our lives, from our physical health to our social interactions, and even our mental well-being.

In this chapter, we'll peel back the layers to uncover the stark realities of obesity and explore the intricate web of factors that contribute to its widespread prevalence.

Exploring Its Consequences

The impact of obesity reverberates far beyond mere numbers on a scale. It's a silent predator lurking within, silently wreaking havoc on our bodies and minds.

Physiologically, obesity sets the stage for a host of chronic diseases, from heart disease to diabetes and everything in between.

It's a heavy burden to carry, not just for individuals but for entire healthcare systems grappling with the staggering costs of treatment and care.

But the consequences of obesity extend far beyond the physical realm. It's a weighty burden that seeps into every corner of our lives, shaping our relationships, our self-esteem, and even our opportunities.

The stigma and shame associated with obesity cast a dark shadow, making it an uphill battle for individuals to find acceptance and support in a society that often equates thinness with worthiness.

Investigating the Triggers Behind the Epidemic

To truly understand the obesity epidemic, we must delve into the tangled web of factors that conspire to fuel its relentless spread. It's a complex interplay of genetics, environment, and lifestyle choices, each thread weaving its own tale of influence.

Genetics may load the gun, but it's our modern environment that pulls the trigger, bombarding us with a constant barrage of unhealthy food options and sedentary lifestyles.

The rise of processed foods, laden with sugars, fats, and empty calories, has transformed the way we eat, eroding traditional dietary patterns and leading us down a dangerous path of weight gain and metabolic dysfunction.

Add to that the pressures of modern life, with its relentless pace and constant stress, and it's no wonder that obesity has become a global epidemic of monumental proportions.

As we navigate the complexities of the obesity epidemic in this chapter, we do so with a sense of urgency and purpose.

It's a call to action, a rallying cry to confront the harsh realities of obesity head-on and forge a path toward a healthier, brighter future.

By shining a light on its consequences and unravelling the intricate web of triggers behind its rise, we arm ourselves with the knowledge and understanding needed to enact meaningful change.

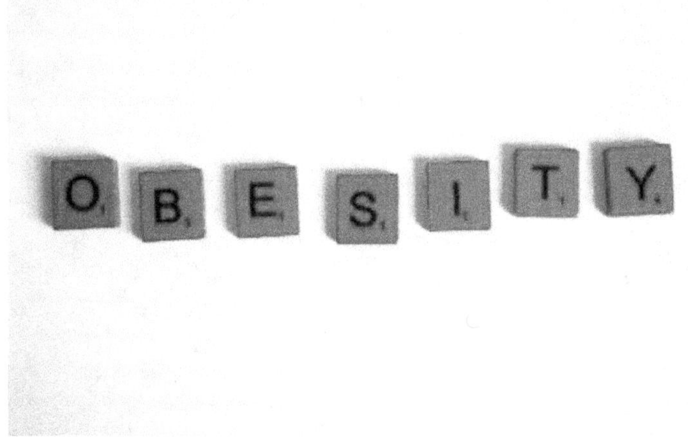

Causes of Obesity

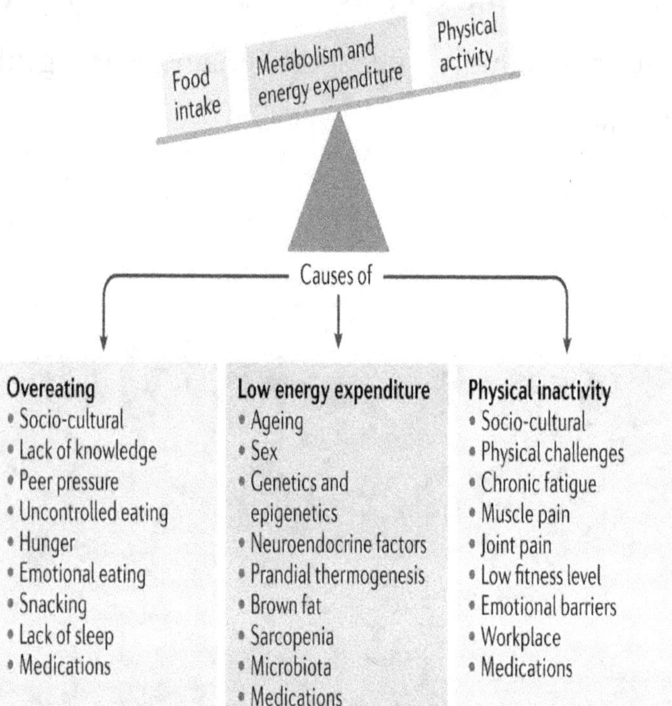

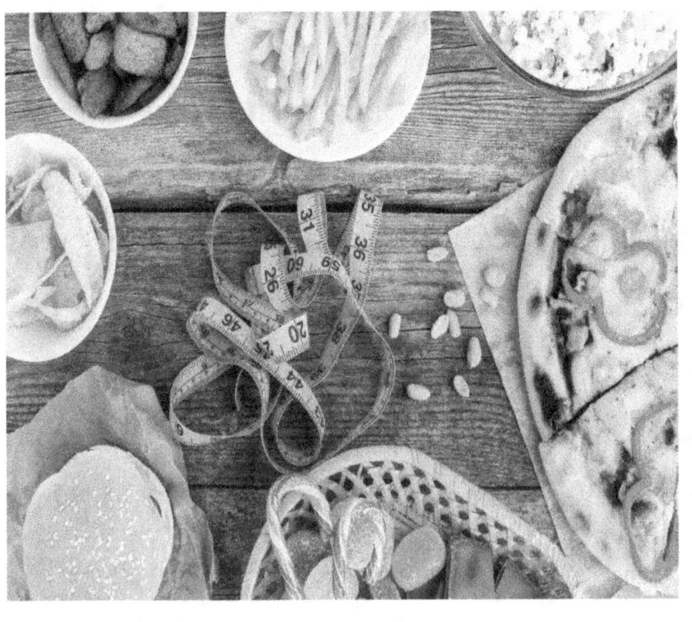

Chapter 2: Demystifying Calories

In our quest to understand the intricate workings of nutrition and weight management, the exploration calories become a journey of revelation and empowerment.

In this chapter, we embark on a voyage to unravel the myths surrounding calories while embracing the scientific realities that underpin energy balance and weight management, offering a balanced perspective accessible to all.

Dissecting Myths and Embracing Scientific Realities

In the realm of nutrition, myths and misconceptions about calories abound, clouding our understanding of their role in our daily lives.

One prevalent myth is the belief that all calories are created equal, implying that the source of calories matters little in the grand scheme of weight management.

However, scientific evidence paints a more nuanced picture, highlighting the importance of nutrient density and overall diet quality in determining metabolic responses and health outcomes.

Another myth to dispel is the notion of "good" and "bad" calories, suggesting that certain foods inherently lead to weight gain while others promote weight loss.

In reality, the impact of calories on weight management is influenced by various factors, including macronutrient composition, fibre content, and individual metabolic differences.

Understanding these complexities allows us to make informed dietary choices that support our health goals.

Understanding Energy Balance and Weight Management

At the heart of weight management lies the concept of energy balance, which dictates that weight stability is achieved when energy intake (calories consumed) equals energy expenditure (calories burned).

This fundamental principle underscores the importance of mindful eating and regular physical activity in achieving and maintaining a healthy weight.

However, achieving energy balance is not solely about counting calories; it's about fostering a holistic approach to nutrition and lifestyle that promotes overall well-being.

This includes prioritizing nutrient-dense foods, practicing portion control, and incorporating regular exercise into our daily routines.

By embracing these scientific realities and dispelling common myths, we empower ourselves to take control of our health and make meaningful changes that support long-term weight management and vitality.

In this chapter, we invite readers to embark on a journey of discovery and empowerment as we unravel the mysteries of calories and embrace the scientific truths that guide us towards a healthier, happier life.

Through a balanced and evidence-based approach, we navigate the complexities of nutrition and weight management with clarity and confidence, laying the foundation for sustainable health and well-being.

Chapter 3: Hormonal Harmony of Obesity Mechanisms

Embarking on an exploration of obesity mechanisms feels akin to diving into the depths of a vast ocean, where the currents of hormones, genetics, and environment converge to shape our body's equilibrium.

In this chapter, we embark on a journey to unravel the intricate interplay of hormones while exploring the genetic and environmental factors that contribute to the obesity epidemic, offering insights and solutions that resonate with readers of all backgrounds.

Unravelling the Intricate Interplay of Hormones

Hormones serve as the body's messengers, orchestrating a symphony of signals that regulate metabolism, hunger, and energy expenditure.

One key player in this symphony is insulin, a hormone secreted by the pancreas in response to food intake. Insulin helps cells absorb glucose from the bloodstream, regulating blood sugar levels and promoting energy storage.

However, in individuals with insulin resistance, cells become less responsive to insulin, leading to elevated blood sugar levels and increased fat storage, particularly in the abdominal region.

Another hormone that influences weight regulation is leptin, often referred to as the "satiety hormone." Leptin is produced by fat cells and signals to the brain when we've had enough to eat, helping to regulate appetite and energy balance.

However, in individuals with obesity, leptin resistance may develop, leading to impaired appetite control and continued overeating.

Exploring Genetic and Environmental Factors

While hormones play a significant role in obesity mechanisms, their effects are modulated by a complex interplay of genetic and environmental factors.

Genetic predispositions can influence an individual's susceptibility to obesity, with certain gene variants predisposing individuals to weight gain and metabolic dysfunction in response to environmental triggers.

Environmental factors, including diet, physical activity, and socio-economic status, also play a crucial role in shaping obesity risk.

The modern obesogenic environment, characterized by an abundance of highly processed, calorie-dense foods and sedentary lifestyles, exacerbates genetic predispositions and contributes to the obesity epidemic.

Understanding the intricate interplay of hormones, genetics, and environment provides valuable insights into obesity mechanisms and informs targeted interventions.

By addressing underlying hormonal imbalances through lifestyle modifications, such as adopting a balanced diet, engaging in regular physical activity, and managing stress levels, individuals can support hormonal harmony and promote healthy weight management.

In this chapter, we have embarked on a deep dive into obesity mechanisms, unravelling the intricate interplay of hormones while exploring genetic and environmental factors.

By providing solutions grounded in scientific evidence and real-world experiences, we empower readers to navigate the complexities of obesity with clarity and confidence, paving the way for sustainable health and well-being.

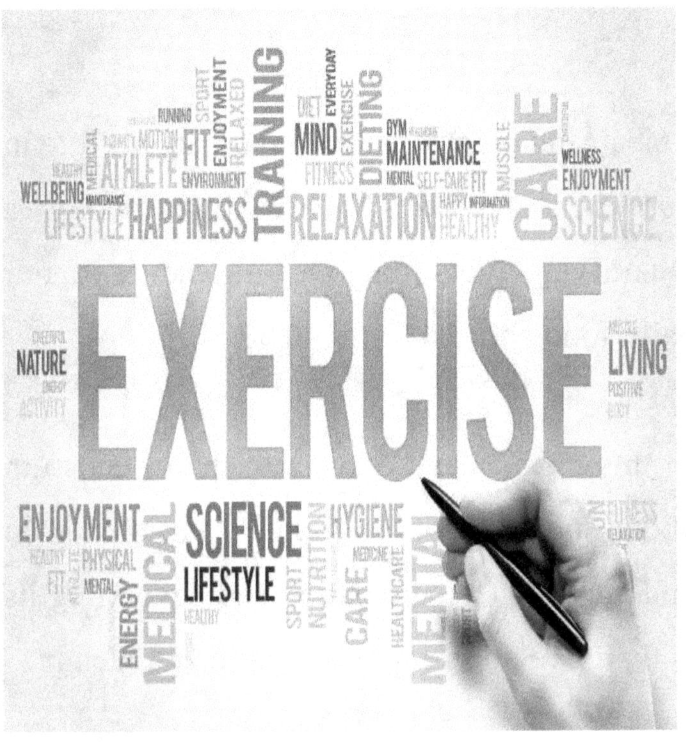

EXERCISE
TRAINING
SPORT
ENJOYMENT
RELAXED
FIT
RUNNING
MOTION
ATHLETE
MEDICAL
HEALTHY
WELLBEING
MAINTENANCE
LIFESTYLE
HAPPINESS
ENVIRONMENT
DIET
EVERYDAY
MIND
EXERCISE
DIETING
FITNESS
MENTAL
SELF-CARE
FIT
GYM
MAINTENANCE
HAPPY
INFORMATION
RELAXATION
HEALTHY
MUSCLE
CARE
WELLNESS
ENJOYMENT
SCIENCE
CHEERFUL
NATURE
ENERGY
ACTIVITY
MUSCLE
LIVING
POSITIVE
BODY
ENJOYMENT
HEALTHY
PHYSICAL
FIT
MENTAL
ATHLETE
MEDICAL
SCIENCE
LIFESTYLE
HEALTHY
ENERGY
SPORT
NUTRITION
HYGIENE
MEDICINE
CARE
HEALTHCARE
MENTAL
FITNESS
RELAXATION

Chapter 4: The Sweet Truth about Sugar

Embarking on an exploration of sugar's role in our diets is akin to peering through a magnifying glass into the intricacies of our daily food choices.

In this chapter, we delve into the sweet truth about sugar, shedding light on its impact on abdominal fat accumulation and navigating its complex relationship with health and weight.

In the modern world, sugar has become ubiquitous, sneaking its way into countless processed foods and beverages.

However, its sweet allure belies a darker reality: excessive sugar consumption is closely linked to abdominal fat accumulation, also known as visceral fat.

This type of fat is not merely a passive storage depot but rather an active endocrine organ that secretes hormones and inflammatory substances, contributing to metabolic dysfunction and increased disease risk.

Research has shown that high sugar intake, particularly in the form of added sugars found in sugary beverages, sweets, and processed foods, is strongly associated with visceral fat deposition.

The fructose component of sugar, in particular, is metabolized in the liver, where it can promote fat synthesis and contribute to the development of fatty liver disease and insulin resistance.

Understanding sugar's impact on health and weight requires a multifaceted approach that considers both its physiological effects and behavioural implications.

From a physiological standpoint, excessive sugar consumption can disrupt metabolic pathways, leading to insulin resistance, inflammation, and dysregulation of appetite hormones.

Behaviourally, sugar's addictive properties can lead to overconsumption, contributing to a cycle of cravings, binge eating, and weight gain.

Breaking free from the grip of sugar addiction requires mindfulness, awareness, and strategies to reduce sugar intake gradually.

Examples of effective strategies include:

- Reading food labels to identify hidden sugars in processed foods.

- Opting for whole, unprocessed foods that are naturally low in added sugars.

- Substituting sugary beverages with water, herbal teas, or infused water.

- Incorporating more fiber-rich foods like fruits, vegetables, and whole grains to promote satiety and stabilize blood sugar levels.

By adopting these strategies and cultivating a balanced approach to sugar consumption, individuals can mitigate the negative effects of excessive sugar intake and promote overall health and well-being.

In this chapter, we have explored the sweet truth about sugar, shedding light on its role in abdominal fat accumulation and navigating its impact on health and weight.

By understanding the physiological and behavioural mechanisms at play, we empower ourselves to make informed dietary choices and cultivate a healthier relationship with sugar.

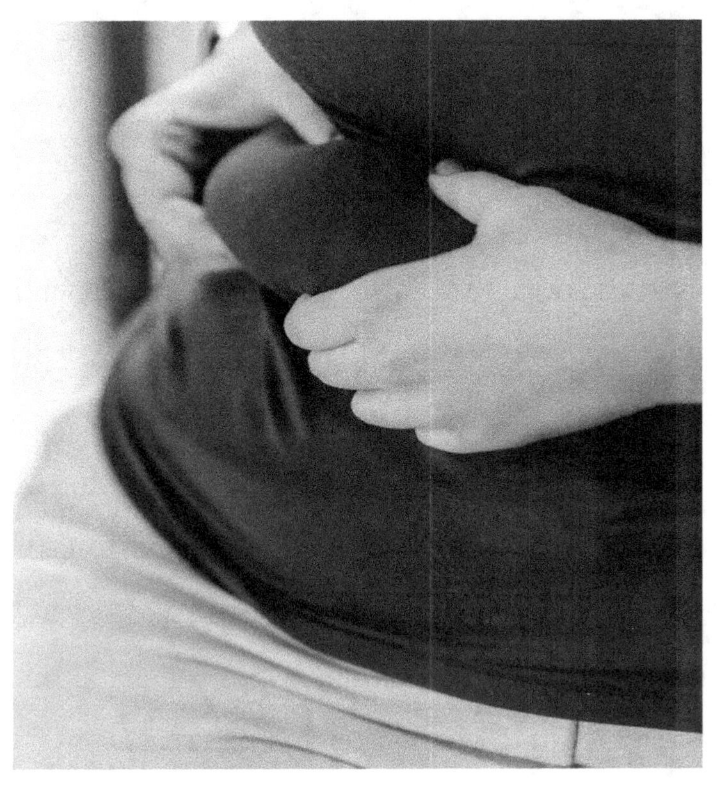

Chapter 5: Flour, Fat, and the Modern Diet

As we navigate the complexities of the modern diet, the roles of refined flour and fats emerge as critical factors influencing our health and weight.

In this chapter, we embark on an exploration of their nuanced impacts, evaluating the role of refined flour in obesity trends and understanding the complexities of fat from weight gain to weight management.

By unravelling these intricacies, we aim to provide readers with actionable insights and solutions to navigate the modern dietary landscape with confidence and clarity.

Evaluating the Role of Refined Flour in Obesity Trends

Refined flour, a staple ingredient in many processed foods, has become ubiquitous in the modern diet. However, its widespread use is not without consequences, particularly in relation to obesity trends.

Refined flour undergoes processing that strips away the outer bran and germ layers, leaving behind a fine, white powder devoid of fibre and essential nutrients.

This refining process results in a product that is rapidly digested and absorbed by the body, leading to sharp spikes in blood sugar levels and subsequent crashes.

These fluctuations in blood sugar can disrupt hunger signals, leading to increased appetite and overeating a phenomenon linked to weight gain and obesity.

Moreover, the consumption of refined flour is often associated with the consumption of other calorie-dense, nutrient-poor foods, further exacerbating the risk of weight gain and metabolic dysfunction.

By evaluating the role of refined flour in obesity trends, we can better understand the importance of reducing its intake and opting for whole, unprocessed alternatives whenever possible.

Understanding the Nuances of Fat: From Weight Gain to Weight Management

In contrast to the demonization of fats in the past, we now recognize that not all fats are created equal.

While certain fats, such as trans fats and excessive saturated fats, have been linked to adverse health outcomes, others play essential roles in our bodies and can even support weight management.

For example, unsaturated fats, found in foods like avocados, nuts, and olive oil, have been shown to have beneficial effects on heart health and may help promote satiety when consumed in moderation.

Additionally, omega-3 fatty acids, found in fatty fish like salmon and mackerel, have anti-inflammatory properties and may support overall well-being.

By understanding the nuances of fat and incorporating healthy fats into our diets, we can optimize our health and support weight management goals.

This includes choosing lean sources of protein, incorporating plant-based fats, and prioritizing whole foods over processed options.

In navigating the complexities of flour and fat in the modern diet, it is essential to prioritize whole, unprocessed foods and to be mindful of portion sizes.

By reducing our intake of refined flour and incorporating healthy fats into our diets, we can support overall health and well-being while mitigating the risk of weight gain and obesity.

By providing practical solutions grounded in scientific evidence, we empower readers to make informed dietary choices and navigate the modern food landscape with confidence.

In doing so, we take a step towards achieving our goal of promoting sustainable health and well-being for all.

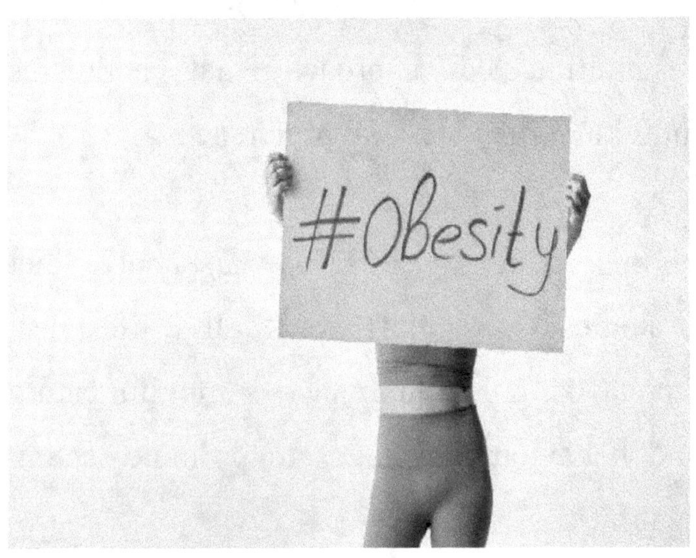

Chapter 6: Crafting Your Path to Health

In our journey towards optimal health and well-being, crafting a sustainable path requires a multifaceted approach that addresses individual lifestyles and preferences.

In this chapter, we explore sustainable diet strategies suitable for all lifestyles, emphasizing the importance of mindful eating and behavioural changes to promote lasting health transformations.

By incorporating these principles into our daily lives, we can cultivate a balanced approach to nutrition and embark on a journey towards lifelong wellness.

Sustainable Diet Strategies for All Lifestyles

Adopting a sustainable diet is not about strict rules or deprivation; rather, it's about finding a balance that works for you and supports your overall health goals.

One approach is to focus on whole, unprocessed foods that nourish the body and provide essential nutrients.

This includes incorporating plenty of fruits, vegetables, whole grains, lean proteins, and healthy fats into your meals.

Another key aspect of a sustainable diet is to practice portion control and mindful eating. By paying attention to hunger and fullness cues, you can avoid overeating and better regulate your food intake.

This may involve slowing down during meals, savouring each bite, and listening to your body's signals of hunger and satiety.

Additionally, it's important to find joy in food and to cultivate a positive relationship with eating. This may involve experimenting with new recipes, enjoying meals with loved ones, and exploring different culinary traditions.

By approaching food with a sense of curiosity and appreciation, you can enhance your overall eating experience and support sustainable dietary habits.

Incorporating Mindful Eating and Behavioural Changes

In addition to adopting sustainable diet strategies, incorporating mindful eating practices and behavioural changes can further support your journey towards health. Mindful eating involves being present and attentive while eating, focusing on the sensory experience of food, and tuning into your body's hunger and fullness cues.

One strategy to practice mindful eating is to engage all your senses while eating, paying attention to the colours, textures, flavours, and aromas of your food.

This can enhance your enjoyment of meals and help you feel more satisfied with smaller portions.

Another approach is to minimize distractions while eating, such as watching TV or using electronic devices, and instead focus on the act of eating and the sensations it brings.

In terms of behavioural changes, it's important to identify and address any habits or patterns that may be contributing to unhealthy eating behaviours.

This may involve keeping a food journal to track your eating habits, identifying triggers for overeating or emotional eating, and developing coping strategies to address these triggers in healthier ways.

By incorporating mindful eating practices and making behavioural changes, you can cultivate a more balanced and sustainable approach to nutrition, supporting your long-term health and well-being.

Examples of sustainable diet strategies and mindful eating practices include:

- Meal planning and preparation to ensure access to nutritious foods throughout the week.

- Setting realistic and achievable goals for healthy eating, such as incorporating more fruits and vegetables into your meals or reducing your intake of processed foods.

- Seeking support from friends, family, or a registered dietitian to help you stay accountable and motivated on your health journey.

In conclusion, crafting your path to health involves adopting sustainable diet strategies tailored to your lifestyle and preferences, as well as incorporating mindful eating practices and behavioural changes to support long-term success.

By embracing these principles and making gradual, sustainable changes, you can achieve lasting health transformations and embark on a journey towards lifelong wellness.

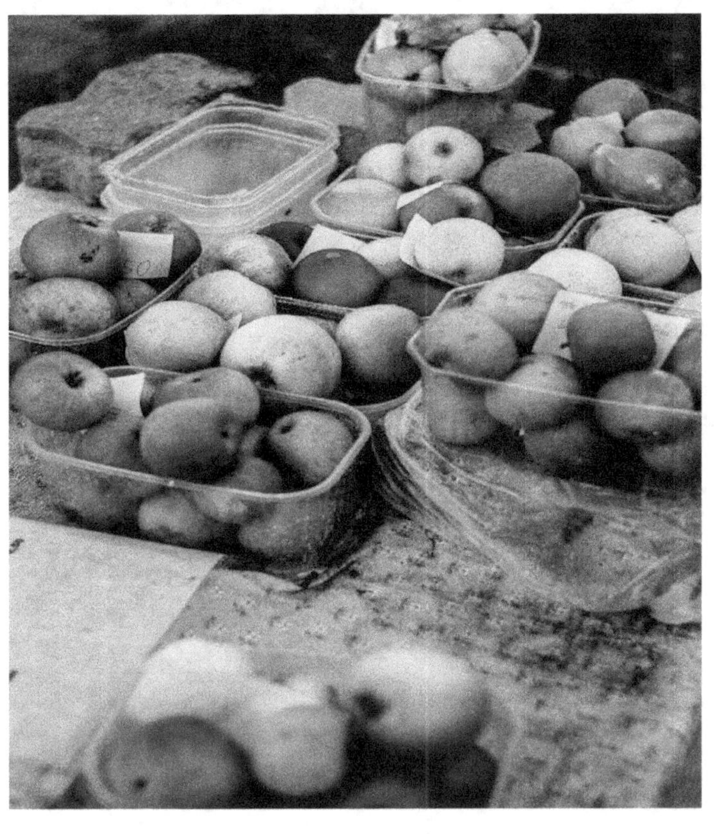

Chapter 7: The Obesity Solution Diet Plan

Embarking on a journey towards sustainable weight loss requires a comprehensive approach that encompasses not only dietary changes but also practical strategies for success.

In this chapter, we present The Obesity Solution Diet Plan a holistic and science-based approach to achieving lasting weight loss.

By providing meal plans, recipes, and practical tips tailored to both science and non-science readers, we aim to empower individuals to take control of their health and embark on a journey towards a healthier, happier life.

A Comprehensive Approach to Sustainable Weight Loss

The Obesity Solution Diet Plan is grounded in the principles of balanced nutrition, mindful eating, and behavioural changes, providing a comprehensive framework for achieving and maintaining a healthy weight.

It emphasizes the importance of whole, unprocessed foods, portion control, and regular physical activity as key components of a sustainable weight loss plan.

Meal Plans and Recipes

The Obesity Solution Diet Plan offers customizable meal plans and recipes designed to meet the diverse needs and preferences of individuals.

These meal plans are based on nutrient-rich foods such as fruits, vegetables, lean proteins, and whole grains, providing a balance of macronutrients and micronutrients essential for optimal health.

Sample meal plans may include:

- Breakfast: Greek yogurt with mixed berries and almonds

- Lunch: Grilled chicken salad with mixed greens, tomatoes, cucumbers, and avocado

- Dinner: Baked salmon with quinoa and roasted vegetables

In addition to meal plans, The Obesity Solution Diet Plan provides a variety of delicious and nutritious recipes that are easy to prepare and incorporate into daily meals.

From hearty soups and salads to flavourful stir-fries and grilled entrees, these recipes offer a diverse range of options to suit different tastes and dietary preferences.

Practical Tips for Success

In addition to meal plans and recipes, The Obesity Solution Diet Plan offers practical tips and strategies to support individuals on their weight loss journey. These tips may include:

- Keeping a food journal to track eating habits and identify areas for improvement.

- Planning meals and snacks ahead of time to avoid impulsive food choices.

- Incorporating physical activity into daily routines, such as walking, biking, or yoga.

- Practicing mindfulness and stress management techniques to reduce emotional eating.

By incorporating these practical tips into daily life, individuals can build sustainable habits that support long-term weight loss and overall health.

In conclusion, The Obesity Solution Diet Plan offers a comprehensive approach to sustainable weight loss, providing meal plans, recipes, and practical tips tailored to both science and non-science readers.

By embracing this holistic approach and making gradual, sustainable changes, individuals can achieve lasting success on their journey towards a healthier, happier life.

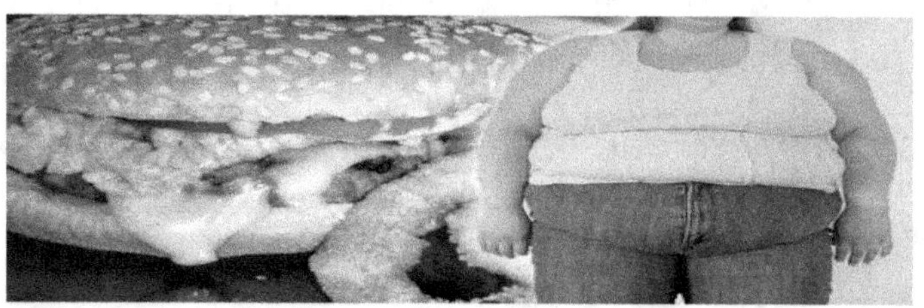

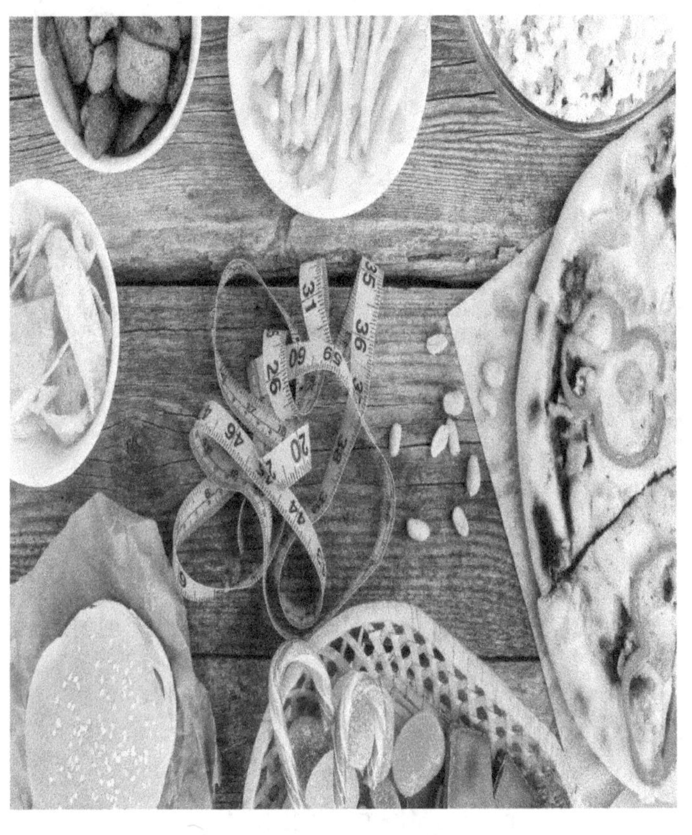

Chapter 8: Beyond Weight Loss: Embracing Health and Vitality

As we journey towards improved health, it's essential to recognize that the benefits of a healthy lifestyle extend far beyond mere weight loss.

In this chapter, we delve into the multifaceted advantages of embracing a holistic approach to health and vitality, exploring how a balanced lifestyle impacts both body and mind.

By understanding these benefits, readers can gain a deeper appreciation for the value of prioritizing their well-being and making sustainable lifestyle changes.

Exploring the Benefits of a Healthy Lifestyle Beyond the Scale

A healthy lifestyle encompasses various facets, including nutritious eating, regular physical activity, adequate sleep, stress management, and social connections.

While weight loss may be a primary goal for many, the benefits of adopting a healthy lifestyle extend beyond mere numbers on the scale.

Improved Physical Health:

One of the most notable benefits of a healthy lifestyle is improved physical health. Regular exercise strengthens the cardiovascular system, boosts immune function, and reduces the risk of chronic diseases such as heart disease, diabetes, and certain cancers.

Additionally, a balanced diet rich in fruits, vegetables, lean proteins, and whole grains provides essential nutrients that support overall health and vitality.

Enhanced Mental Well-being:

In addition to physical health, a healthy lifestyle has profound effects on mental well-being. Regular physical activity releases endorphins, neurotransmitters that promote feelings of happiness and reduce stress and anxiety.

Adequate sleep and stress management techniques, such as mindfulness and relaxation exercises, further support mental health and resilience in the face of life's challenges.

Increased Energy and Vitality:
By nourishing the body with wholesome foods and engaging in regular physical activity,

individuals experience increased energy levels and vitality.

This heightened sense of well-being enables them to tackle daily tasks with vigour and enthusiasm, enhancing overall productivity and quality of life.

Improved Quality of Life:

Ultimately, the benefits of embracing a healthy lifestyle translate into an improved quality of life. Whether it's enjoying outdoor activities with loved ones, pursuing hobbies and interests, or simply feeling more confident and comfortable in one's own skin, a balanced approach to health and vitality enriches every aspect of life.

Solutions and Practical Tips

To embrace health and vitality beyond weight loss, individuals can incorporate various lifestyle practices into their daily routines. These may include:

- Engaging in regular physical activity, such as walking, jogging, cycling, or yoga.

- Prioritizing sleep hygiene and aiming for seven to eight hours of quality sleep each night.

- Practicing stress management techniques, such as deep breathing exercises, meditation, or spending time in nature.

- Nourishing the body with a balanced diet rich in fruits, vegetables, whole grains, lean proteins, and healthy fats.

- Cultivating social connections and maintaining supportive relationships with friends and family.

By integrating these practices into their lives, individuals can experience the multifaceted benefits of a healthy lifestyle, ultimately achieving greater health, vitality, and overall well-being.

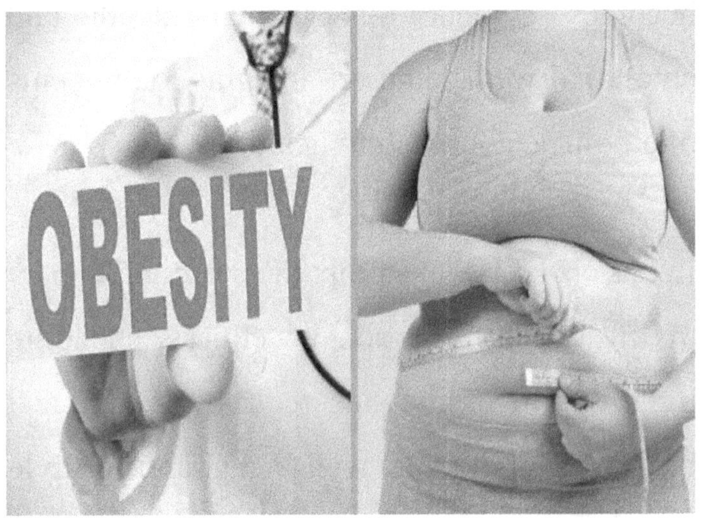

Chapter 9: Mental Health and Emotional Well-Being

As we delve into the intricate web of lifestyle factors that impact our overall well-being, it becomes evident that mental health and emotional well-being are integral components of a holistic approach to health.

In this chapter, we explore the profound impact of lifestyle on emotional wellness, shedding light on the interconnectedness of physical health, psychological well-being, and lifestyle choices.

By understanding these relationships and implementing strategies to support mental health, readers can cultivate resilience, emotional balance, and overall life satisfaction.

Exploring the Profound Impact of Lifestyle on Emotional Wellness

The relationship between lifestyle and emotional wellness is multifaceted and dynamic, encompassing various factors such as diet, physical activity, sleep, stress management, social connections, and self-care practices.

Each of these elements plays a crucial role in shaping our mental health and emotional well-being, highlighting the importance of adopting a comprehensive approach to self-care.

Diet:

Nutrition plays a significant role in mental health, with research indicating that certain dietary patterns are associated with a lower risk of depression and anxiety.

A diet rich in fruits, vegetables, whole grains, lean proteins, and healthy fats provides essential nutrients that support brain function and mood regulation.

Additionally, reducing the intake of processed foods, sugary beverages, and artificial additives can help stabilize mood and promote emotional well-being.

Physical Activity:

Regular physical activity has been shown to have profound effects on mental health, reducing symptoms of depression, anxiety, and stress while improving mood and overall well-being.

Engaging in activities such as walking, jogging, swimming, or yoga not only boosts endorphin levels but also enhances self-esteem, cognitive function, and emotional resilience.

Sleep:

Quality sleep is essential for emotional regulation and mental health, with inadequate sleep linked to increased risk of mood disorders and cognitive impairment.

Prioritizing good sleep hygiene practices, such as maintaining a regular sleep schedule, creating a relaxing bedtime routine, and creating a conducive sleep environment, can promote restful sleep and support emotional well-being.

Stress Management:

Chronic stress can have detrimental effects on mental health, contributing to anxiety, depression, and other mood disorders.

Effective stress management techniques, such as mindfulness meditation, deep breathing exercises, progressive muscle relaxation, and engaging in hobbies and activities that bring joy, can help reduce stress levels and enhance emotional resilience.

Social Connections:

Social connections and supportive relationships are fundamental to emotional well-being, providing a sense of belonging, acceptance, and validation.

Nurturing friendships, cultivating community ties, and seeking support from loved ones during challenging times can bolster mental health and provide a vital source of emotional support.

Self-Care Practices:
Incorporating self-care practices into daily life is essential for maintaining emotional well-being and preventing burnout.

This may include setting aside time for relaxation and leisure activities, practicing self-compassion and self-acceptance, setting boundaries, and prioritizing activities that promote personal growth and fulfilment.

Solutions and Practical Tips

To support mental health and emotional well-being, individuals can incorporate various lifestyle practices into their daily routines. These may include:

- Prioritizing nutritious meals that support brain health and mood regulation.

- Engaging in regular physical activity to boost endorphin levels and promote emotional resilience.

- Establishing healthy sleep habits and creating a conducive sleep environment to ensure restful sleep.

- Practicing stress management techniques, such as mindfulness meditation and deep breathing exercises, to reduce stress levels.

- Cultivating social connections and seeking support from loved ones during challenging times.

- Incorporating self-care practices into daily life to nurture emotional well-being and prevent burnout.

By integrating these strategies into their lives, individuals can support their mental health and emotional well-being, cultivate resilience, and enhance overall life satisfaction.

In conclusion, the profound impact of lifestyle on emotional wellness underscores the importance of adopting a comprehensive approach to self-care.

By prioritizing nutrition, physical activity, sleep, stress management, social connections, and self-care practices, individuals can support their mental health and emotional well-being, cultivate resilience, and enhance overall life satisfaction.

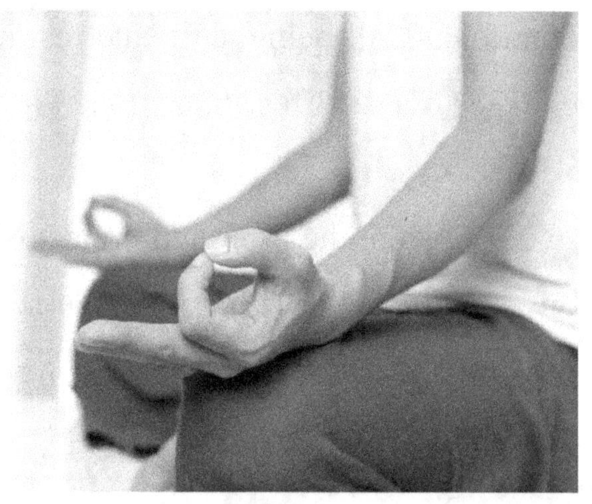

20-Minute Yoga Workout for Beginners

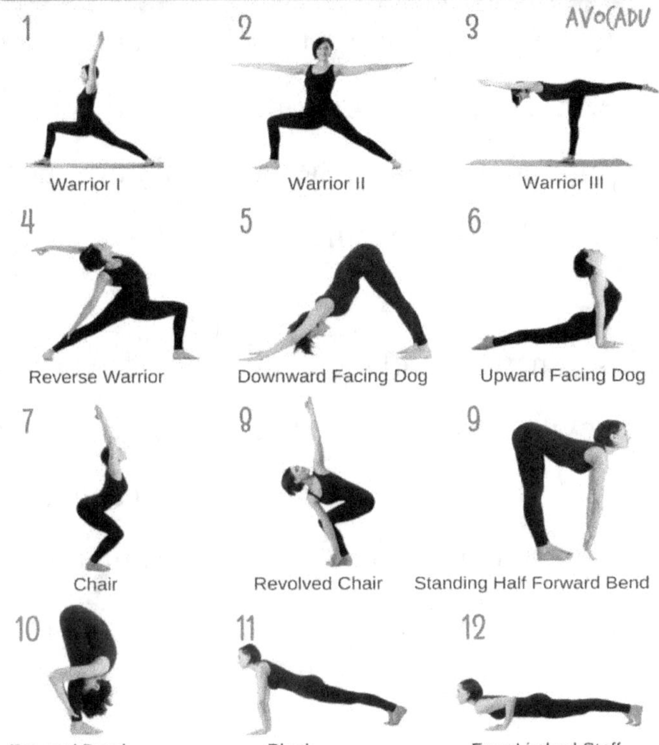

Chapter 10: Longevity and Aging

Unlocking the Secrets to a Longer, Healthier Life in the pursuit of longevity and graceful aging, understanding the factors that influence our health span becomes paramount.

This chapter delves into the science of longevity and aging, shedding light on the intricate interplay of genetic, lifestyle, and environmental factors that shape our lifespan and quality of life.

By uncovering the secrets to a longer, healthier life, readers can gain valuable insights and practical strategies to optimize their well-being and embrace the aging process with vitality and resilience.

Exploring the Science of Longevity

Longevity, the art of living a long and fulfilling life, is influenced by a myriad of factors that extend beyond mere genetics. While genetics certainly play a role in determining our lifespan, emerging research suggests that lifestyle choices and environmental factors exert a significant influence on our health span the number of years we live in good health.

Genetic Factors:

Our genes provide a blueprint for our health and longevity, influencing factors such as metabolism, cellular repair mechanisms, and susceptibility to age-related diseases.

However, it's essential to recognize that genetics are not destiny; lifestyle choices can modulate gene expression and impact our health outcomes.

Lifestyle Factors:

Adopting healthy lifestyle habits is paramount for promoting longevity and healthy aging. These include:

- Maintaining a balanced diet rich in fruits, vegetables, whole grains, lean proteins, and healthy fats.

- Engaging in regular physical activity to support cardiovascular health, muscle strength, and overall well-being.

- Prioritizing sleep and stress management to optimize restorative sleep and reduce the detrimental effects of chronic stress.

- Nurturing social connections and maintaining meaningful relationships to foster emotional resilience and mental well-being

- Incorporating brain-boosting activities such as mental stimulation, lifelong learning, and social engagement to support cognitive health.

Environmental Factors:

Environmental factors, such as exposure to pollutants, toxins, and lifestyle choices, can impact our health and longevity.

Minimizing exposure to harmful substances, prioritizing clean air and water, and making conscious choices that support environmental sustainability can contribute to overall well-being and longevity.

In addition to understanding the factors that influence longevity, implementing practical strategies can further support healthy aging and vitality:

Prioritizing preventive healthcare, including regular check-ups, screenings, and vaccinations, to detect and address potential health issues early.

Embracing positive lifestyle changes, such as quitting smoking, limiting alcohol consumption, and avoiding excessive sun exposure, to reduce the risk of chronic diseases and premature aging.

Cultivating a sense of purpose and meaning in life, whether through hobbies, volunteer work, or creative pursuits, to promote psychological well-being and resilience.

Adopting a flexible mind-set and embracing life's transitions with grace and adaptability, recognizing that aging is a natural and inevitable part of the human experience.

By unlocking the secrets to a longer, healthier life and implementing practical strategies for longevity, individuals can optimize their health span and embrace the aging process with vitality, resilience, and grace.

In conclusion, longevity and aging are influenced by a complex interplay of genetic, lifestyle, and environmental factors.

By understanding these factors and implementing practical strategies for healthy aging, individuals can unlock the secrets to a longer, healthier life and embrace the aging process with vitality and resilience.

Chapter 11: Disease Prevention and Management

Harnessing the Power of Lifestyle Medicine for Better Health in our quest for optimal health and well-being, understanding the role of lifestyle medicine in disease prevention and management is paramount.

This chapter explores the transformative potential of lifestyle interventions in mitigating the risk of chronic diseases, managing existing health conditions, and promoting overall wellness.

By harnessing the power of lifestyle medicine, individuals can take proactive steps to optimize their health and live vibrant, fulfilling lives.

The Impact of Lifestyle on Disease Prevention

Lifestyle factors, including diet, physical activity, sleep, stress management, and social connections, play a pivotal role in preventing a myriad of chronic diseases, including heart disease, diabetes, obesity, cancer, and mental health disorders.

By adopting healthy lifestyle habits, individuals can significantly reduce their risk of developing these conditions and promote longevity and well-being.

Diet:

A balanced and nutritious diet is foundational to disease prevention and management.

Emphasizing whole, unprocessed foods such as fruits, vegetables, whole grains, lean proteins, and healthy fats can help maintain a healthy weight, regulate blood sugar levels, support cardiovascular health, and reduce inflammation all of which are crucial for preventing chronic diseases.

Physical Activity:

Regular physical activity is a cornerstone of disease prevention, with numerous studies demonstrating its benefits for cardiovascular health, metabolic function, mental well-being, and overall longevity.

Engaging in activities such as brisk walking, cycling, swimming, or strength training can help maintain a healthy weight, strengthen muscles and bones, improve mood, and reduce the risk of chronic diseases.

Sleep:

Quality sleep is essential for overall health and well-being, playing a crucial role in immune function, cognitive function, mood regulation, and hormone balance.

Prioritizing good sleep hygiene practices, such as maintaining a consistent sleep schedule, creating a comfortable sleep environment, and practicing relaxation techniques, can support optimal health and reduce the risk of chronic diseases.

Stress Management:

Chronic stress can have detrimental effects on physical and mental health, contributing to the development and progression of various chronic diseases.

Incorporating stress management techniques such as mindfulness meditation, deep breathing exercises, yoga, or spending time in nature can help mitigate the impact of stress and promote overall well-being.

Social Connections:

Strong social connections and supportive relationships are associated with better health outcomes, including reduced risk of chronic diseases and improved mental well-being.

Nurturing friendships, participating in community activities, and seeking support from loved ones during challenging times can enhance resilience and promote overall health and longevity.

Practical Strategies for Disease Prevention and Management

In addition to understanding the impact of lifestyle on disease prevention, implementing practical strategies can further support optimal health and well-being: Establishing realistic and achievable health goals based on individual needs and preferences.

Seeking guidance from healthcare professionals, such as doctors, dietitians, and fitness experts, to develop personalized lifestyle plans.

Making gradual and sustainable changes to diet, physical activity, sleep, and stress management habits to promote long-term success.

Incorporating social support and accountability mechanisms, such as joining a fitness class, participating in a support group, or enlisting the help of a workout buddy, to stay motivated and on track.

By harnessing the power of lifestyle medicine and adopting proactive strategies for disease prevention and management, individuals can take control of their health destiny and pave the way for a vibrant, fulfilling life.

In conclusion, lifestyle medicine offers a holistic and empowering approach to disease prevention and management, emphasizing the transformative potential of healthy lifestyle habits in optimizing health and well-being.

By prioritizing nutrition, physical activity, sleep, stress management, and social connections, individuals can unlock the power of lifestyle medicine and embark on a journey towards better health and vitality.

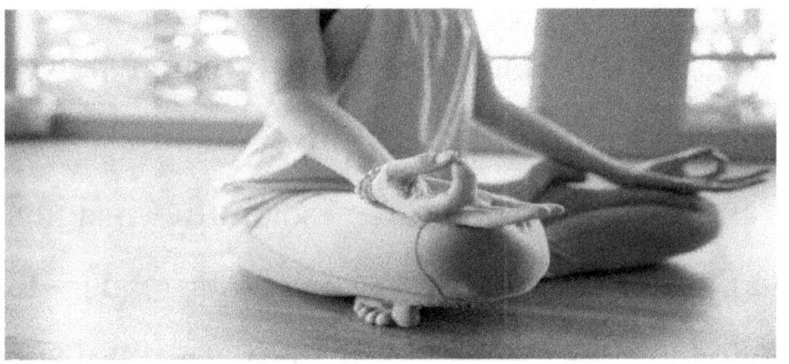

Chapter 12: Holistic Health Approaches

Embracing Mind-Body Practices for Total Well-being in our pursuit of optimal health and well-being, it's essential to embrace holistic approaches that address the interconnectedness of the mind, body, and spirit.

This chapter explores the transformative power of mind-body practices in promoting total well-being, incorporating scientific insights and practical strategies to empower readers to enhance their health from a holistic perspective.

By embracing these holistic health approaches, individuals can cultivate a deeper sense of balance, vitality, and harmony in their lives.

Understanding Holistic Health

Holistic health approaches recognize that optimal well-being is not merely the absence of disease but rather a state of balance and harmony within the body, mind, and spirit.

These approaches acknowledge the interconnectedness of various aspects of life, including physical health, mental and emotional well-being, social connections, and spiritual fulfilment.

By addressing these interconnected factors, individuals can promote total well-being and enhance their overall quality of life.

Mind-Body Practices:

Mind-body practices encompass a wide range of techniques and therapies that promote the integration of mind, body, and spirit to support health and healing.

These practices draw upon ancient wisdom traditions as well as modern scientific research, offering holistic approaches to addressing physical, mental, and emotional health concerns. Some key mind-body practices include:

Meditation:

Meditation involves the practice of focused attention or mindfulness to cultivate inner peace, relaxation, and mental clarity.

Research has shown that regular meditation practice can reduce stress, improve mood, enhance immune function, and promote overall well-being.

Yoga:

Yoga is a mind-body practice that combines physical postures, breath work, and meditation to promote flexibility, strength, and relaxation.

Yoga has been found to have numerous health benefits, including improved cardiovascular health, reduced anxiety and depression, and enhanced overall quality of life.

Tai Chi and Qigong:

Tai Chi and Qigong are ancient Chinese martial arts practices that emphasize slow, gentle movements, coordinated with deep breathing and mindfulness.

These practices have been shown to improve balance, flexibility, and cognitive function, reduce stress, and promote relaxation.

Breath work:

Breath work techniques involve conscious control of the breath to promote relaxation, stress reduction, and emotional well-being.

Deep breathing exercises, such as diaphragmatic breathing and alternate nostril breathing, can help regulate the autonomic nervous system, reduce anxiety, and promote a sense of calm.

Mindfulness-Based Stress Reduction (MBSR):

MBSR is a structured program that combines mindfulness meditation, body awareness, and yoga to help individuals manage stress, pain, and illness. Research has demonstrated the effectiveness of MBSR in reducing stress, improving mood, and enhancing overall well-being.

Practical Strategies for Embracing Holistic Health

Incorporating mind-body practices into daily life can support total well-being and enhance overall quality of life.

Some practical strategies for embracing holistic health include:

- Setting aside time each day for meditation, yoga, or other mind-body practices.

- Participating in classes or workshops to learn new mind-body techniques and deepen your practice.

- Creating a calming and nurturing environment for relaxation and self-care at home. Connecting with nature through outdoor activities, such as hiking, gardening, or simply spending time in natural settings.

- Nurturing social connections and seeking support from friends, family, or community groups. Cultivating gratitude and mindfulness in daily life, focusing on the present moment and appreciating the simple joys and blessings.

By embracing these holistic health approaches and integrating mind-body practices into daily life, individuals can promote total well-being, enhance resilience, and cultivate a deeper sense of balance, vitality, and harmony in their lives.

In conclusion, holistic health approaches offer transformative strategies for promoting total well-being by addressing the interconnectedness of the mind, body, and spirit.

By embracing mind-body practices and incorporating holistic health principles into daily life, individuals can enhance their health from a holistic perspective and cultivate a deeper sense of balance, vitality, and harmony.

Chapter 13: Questions and Answers

What are some current theories on the causes of obesity?

Current theories on the causes of obesity encompass a multifaceted understanding that integrates genetic, environmental, behavioural, and socioeconomic factors.

One prevailing theory is the energy balance model, which suggests that obesity results from an imbalance between energy intake (calories consumed) and energy expenditure (calories burned).

This imbalance can be influenced by various factors, including dietary habits, physical activity levels, metabolic rate, and genetic predispositions.

Another theory focuses on the role of environmental factors, such as the availability and accessibility of high-calorie, processed foods, and the prevalence of sedentary lifestyles.

The obesogenic environment theory posits that modern environments promote excessive calorie consumption and discourage physical activity, contributing to weight gain and obesity.

Additionally, hormonal and metabolic factors play a significant role in the development of obesity. Hormones like insulin, leptin, and ghrelin regulate appetite, metabolism, and fat storage, and dysregulation of these hormones can lead to weight gain and obesity.

Genetic predispositions also play a role, with certain genetic variations influencing metabolism, fat distribution, and susceptibility to obesity.

Psychological and behavioural factors, including stress, emotional eating, and food addiction, are also implicated in the development of obesity.

Socioeconomic factors, such as income level, education, and access to healthcare, can influence dietary choices, physical activity levels, and obesity prevalence.

Overall, obesity is a complex and multifactorial condition influenced by a combination of genetic, environmental, behavioural, and socioeconomic factors. Understanding these diverse influences is essential for developing effective strategies for obesity prevention and management.

Can PFAS cause obesity?

PFAS, or per- and polyfluoroalkyl substances, are a group of synthetic chemicals widely used in various industrial and consumer products for their water- and grease-repellent properties.

While there is ongoing research on the health effects of PFAS exposure, current evidence suggests that these chemicals may contribute to obesity through several mechanisms.

Firstly, PFAS exposure has been associated with metabolic disturbances, including insulin resistance and dyslipidaemia, which are risk factors for obesity.

Studies have shown that higher levels of PFAS in the blood are correlated with increased body mass index (BMI) and waist circumference, suggesting a potential link between PFAS exposure and obesity.

Secondly, PFAS chemicals have been found to disrupt endocrine function and alter hormone regulation, which can affect metabolism and energy balance.

For example, PFAS exposure has been linked to disruptions in thyroid hormone levels, which play a crucial role in regulating metabolism and energy expenditure. Furthermore, PFAS exposure may also influence appetite regulation and food intake.

Animal studies have demonstrated that exposure to certain PFAS chemicals can lead to increased food consumption and weight gain, potentially contributing to obesity development.

While the exact mechanisms by which PFAS contribute to obesity are still being elucidated, emerging evidence suggests that these chemicals may indeed play a role in the obesity epidemic.

However, it's important to note that obesity is a complex condition influenced by multiple factors, and PFAS exposure is just one of many potential contributors.

To mitigate the potential health risks associated with PFAS exposure, individuals can take steps to reduce their exposure to these chemicals.

This can include avoiding products containing PFAS, such as non-stick cookware, waterproof clothing, and certain food packaging materials, and opting for PFAS-free alternatives whenever possible.

Additionally, policymakers and regulatory agencies can implement measures to restrict the use of PFAS in consumer products and industrial processes to protect public health.

Does a lack of sun exposure make you obese?

The relationship between sun exposure and obesity is multifaceted, involving various biological and environmental factors.

While sunlight exposure is essential for vitamin D synthesis, which plays a role in regulating metabolism and weight management, its direct impact on obesity is less clear-cut.

One potential mechanism linking sun exposure and obesity is through the regulation of circadian rhythms. Sunlight exposure helps regulate the body's internal clock, influencing sleep-wake cycles and various physiological processes, including metabolism.

Disruptions in circadian rhythms, such as those caused by insufficient sunlight exposure, have been associated with metabolic disturbances and increased risk of obesity.

Additionally, sunlight exposure may indirectly influence obesity risk through its effects on physical activity levels.

Individuals who spend more time outdoors, exposed to sunlight, may be more physically active, which can contribute to weight management and reduce the risk of obesity.

On the other hand, limited sunlight exposure may be associated with certain lifestyle factors that increase obesity risk.

For example, individuals who spend less time outdoors may be more sedentary and have poorer dietary habits, which can contribute to weight gain and obesity.

It's important to note that while sunlight exposure is essential for overall health and well-being, excessive exposure to sunlight, especially without adequate protection, can increase the risk of skin cancer and other health issues.

Therefore, achieving a balance between sun exposure for vitamin D synthesis and sun protection measures is crucial for maintaining optimal health.

Overall, while there is some evidence suggesting a potential link between inadequate sunlight exposure and obesity risk, the relationship is complex and influenced by various factors.

Further research is needed to better understand the role of sunlight exposure in obesity development and identify effective strategies for prevention and management.

Do you think expanding Medicare coverage to include weight loss drugs would be a cost-effective solution for treating obesity?

Expanding Medicare coverage to include weight loss drugs is a complex issue that requires careful consideration of both the potential benefits and challenges.

While weight loss drugs may offer a promising treatment option for obesity, there are several factors to consider in determining whether this would be a cost-effective solution.

One consideration is the efficacy of weight loss drugs in achieving meaningful and sustained weight loss.

While some weight loss drugs have been shown to be effective in helping individuals lose weight in clinical trials, the real-world effectiveness may vary due to factors such as adherence to medication regimens, individual responses to treatment, and potential side effects.

Additionally, the cost of weight loss drugs and their long-term impact on healthcare spending must be carefully evaluated.

Weight loss drugs can be expensive, and expanding Medicare coverage to include these medications could result in significant healthcare costs.

It's essential to weigh the potential cost savings from reducing obesity-related healthcare expenses against the expenses of providing coverage for weight loss drugs.

Furthermore, addressing obesity requires a comprehensive approach that includes lifestyle interventions, behavioural therapy, and access to resources for healthy eating and physical activity.

While weight loss drugs may be a valuable component of obesity treatment for some individuals, they should be used as part of a broader strategy that addresses the underlying factors contributing to obesity.

Ultimately, the decision to expand Medicare coverage to include weight loss drugs should be based on a thorough assessment of their cost-effectiveness, efficacy, and impact on overall health outcomes.

Further research and evaluation are needed to determine the most appropriate and sustainable approaches to addressing obesity within the healthcare system.

Why does obesity cause snoring?

Obesity is closely linked to snoring due to several physiological factors that are exacerbated by excess body weight. When individuals are overweight or obese, they often have increased fat deposition around the neck and throat area.

This excess fat can lead to the narrowing of the airway, which can obstruct airflow during sleep, causing vibrations in the tissues of the throat and resulting in snoring.

Moreover, individuals with obesity may also have increased amounts of soft tissue in the throat, including the tongue and the soft palate. This excess tissue can further contribute to airway obstruction and snoring.

Additionally, obesity is associated with changes in respiratory function, including decreased lung volume and reduced respiratory muscle strength. These changes can lead to decreased airflow during sleep, contributing to snoring.

Furthermore, obesity is a risk factor for obstructive sleep apnoea (OSA), a sleep disorder characterized by repeated episodes of complete or partial airway obstruction during sleep.

OSA is a significant cause of snoring, and individuals with obesity are at a higher risk of developing this condition due to the factors mentioned above.

Overall, obesity can cause snoring through multiple mechanisms, including increased fat deposition around the neck and throat, excess soft tissue in the throat, changes in respiratory function, and the development of obstructive sleep apnoea.

Addressing obesity through weight loss and lifestyle modifications can help reduce snoring and improve overall sleep quality and respiratory health.

Is there a correlation between being fat and snoring? Why or how?

Yes, there is a correlation between being overweight or obese and snoring, and this correlation is primarily due to the physiological effects of excess body weight on the respiratory system.

When individuals are overweight or obese, they often have increased fat deposition around the neck and throat area.

This excess fat can lead to the narrowing of the airway, which can obstruct airflow during sleep and result in snoring. The increased pressure on the airway caused by excess fat can also lead to the collapse of soft tissues in the throat, further contributing to snoring.

Moreover, individuals with obesity may have increased amounts of soft tissue in the throat, including the tongue and the soft palate. This excess tissue can obstruct the airway during sleep, leading to vibrations in the tissues of the throat and resulting in snoring.

Additionally, obesity is associated with changes in respiratory function, including decreased lung volume and reduced respiratory muscle strength. These changes can lead to decreased airflow during sleep, contributing to snoring.

Furthermore, obesity is a significant risk factor for obstructive sleep apnoea (OSA), a sleep disorder characterized by repeated episodes of complete or partial airway obstruction during sleep. OSA is a major cause of snoring, and individuals with obesity are at a higher risk of developing this condition due to the factors mentioned above.

Overall, the correlation between being overweight or obese and snoring is due to the physiological effects of excess body weight on the respiratory system, including airway narrowing, increased soft tissue in the throat, changes in respiratory function, and the development of obstructive sleep apnoea.

Addressing obesity through weight loss and lifestyle modifications can help reduce snoring and improve overall sleep quality and respiratory health.

What makes someone's voice deep and husky, what are some causes of this condition if it's not due to obesity or smoking habits?

A deep and husky voice can result from various factors, including physiological characteristics, hormonal influences, and environmental factors. While obesity and smoking habits are common causes of a deep and husky voice, there are other potential reasons for this condition.

One possible cause is hormonal influences, particularly during puberty. During this time, hormonal changes can lead to the growth and thickening of the vocal cords, resulting in a deeper voice in both males and females.

This natural physiological process accounts for the deepening of the voice commonly observed during adolescence.

Genetic factors can also play a role in determining vocal characteristics, including the depth and huskiness of the voice. Individuals may inherit specific vocal cord characteristics from their parents, leading to a naturally deeper or huskier voice.

Additionally, certain medical conditions or anatomical abnormalities can contribute to a deep and husky voice.

For example, conditions affecting the thyroid gland, such as hypothyroidism or thyroid nodules, can lead to changes in vocal cord function and voice quality.

Similarly, conditions affecting the larynx or vocal cords, such as vocal cord paralysis or vocal cord nodules, can also result in a deep and husky voice.

Furthermore, environmental factors such as frequent exposure to dry or dusty environments, excessive vocal strain, or vocal abuse can affect voice quality and contribute to a deep and husky voice.

Overall, while obesity and smoking habits are common causes of a deep and husky voice, other factors such as hormonal influences, genetic factors, medical conditions, anatomical abnormalities, and environmental factors can also play a role.

Identifying the underlying cause of a deep and husky voice often requires a thorough evaluation by a healthcare professional, including a medical history, physical examination, and possibly diagnostic tests.

Treatment options will depend on the specific cause of the condition and may include lifestyle modifications, vocal therapy, or medical interventions as appropriate.

Am I obese even though I look overweight, I weigh 225 pounds and I'm 5'9". I don't look like I am covered in fat, just overweight. Am I obese or overweight?

Based on your height and weight, with a body mass index (BMI) calculation, you fall into the category of obesity. Obesity is determined by a BMI of 30 or higher.

However, it's essential to recognize that BMI is a screening tool and doesn't directly measure body fat percentage or distribution.

Even though you may not appear to be "covered in fat," excess weight can still impact your health. It's essential to consider other factors such as muscle mass, body composition, and overall health status.

Additionally, individual perceptions of weight and body image can vary. Being overweight or obese increases the risk of various health conditions, including heart disease, type 2 diabetes, high blood pressure, and certain cancers.

Therefore, regardless of how you perceive your weight, it's crucial to prioritize your health and well-being. Consulting with a healthcare professional can provide a comprehensive assessment of your health status, including discussions about weight management, lifestyle modifications, and potential health risks associated with excess weight.

Remember that achieving and maintaining a healthy weight involves a holistic approach that includes balanced nutrition, regular physical activity, and overall well-being.

What is the highest class of obesity?

The highest class of obesity is known as Class III obesity, also referred to as severe or morbid obesity. This classification is determined based on body mass index (BMI), which is a measure of an individual's weight in relation to their height. Class III obesity is defined as having a BMI of 40 or higher.

Individuals with Class III obesity face significant health risks and challenges compared to those with lower levels of obesity.

The excess weight in this category can lead to various serious health conditions, including heart disease, type 2 diabetes, hypertension, sleep apnoea, certain cancers, and reduced life expectancy.

Managing Class III obesity often requires comprehensive and multidisciplinary approaches, including lifestyle modifications, dietary changes, increased physical activity, behavioural interventions, and in some cases, medical or surgical interventions.

It's essential for individuals with Class III obesity to seek support from healthcare professionals to address their weight-related concerns and improve their overall health and well-being.

Why is there a stigma around obesity despite it being considered a medical condition?

The stigma surrounding obesity persists despite it being recognized as a medical condition due to several complex factors deeply ingrained in societal attitudes and perceptions.

One primary reason for this stigma is the widespread misconception that obesity is solely a result of personal choices and lack of willpower, rather than considering its multifactorial nature involving genetic, environmental, and physiological factors.

Media portrayal and societal norms often perpetuate stereotypes and negative attitudes toward individuals with obesity, leading to discrimination and bias in various aspects of life, including employment, healthcare, education, and interpersonal relationships.

This stigma can have detrimental effects on the mental and emotional well-being of individuals affected by obesity, further exacerbating the issue.

Moreover, there is a prevailing cultural emphasis on thinness as an ideal body type, which reinforces the notion that obesity is undesirable and indicative of personal failure.

This cultural bias can contribute to the marginalization and discrimination experienced by individuals living with obesity.

Addressing the stigma surrounding obesity requires a multifaceted approach involving education, advocacy, and policy changes to promote understanding, empathy, and support for individuals affected by this medical condition.

By challenging stereotypes, promoting body positivity, and fostering inclusive environments, we can work towards reducing the stigma associated with obesity and supporting individuals in achieving their health and wellness goals.

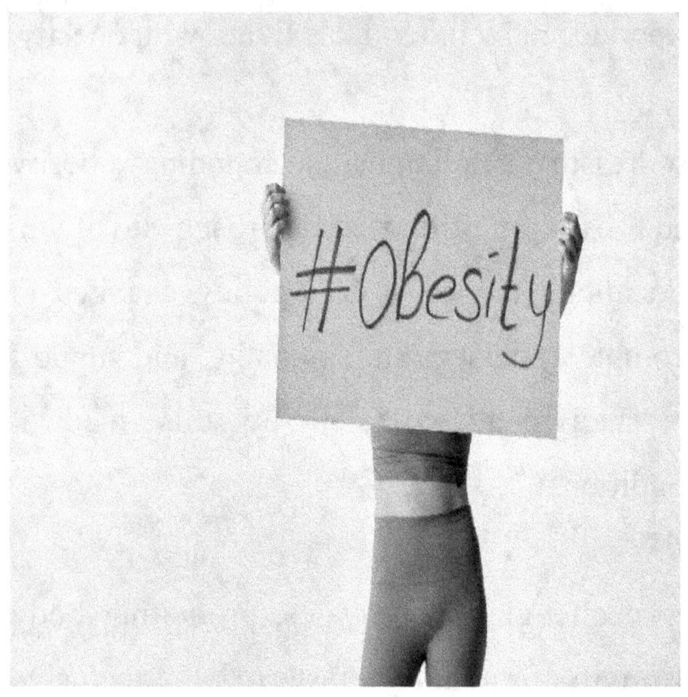

20-MINUTE YOGA WORKOUT FOR BEGINNERS

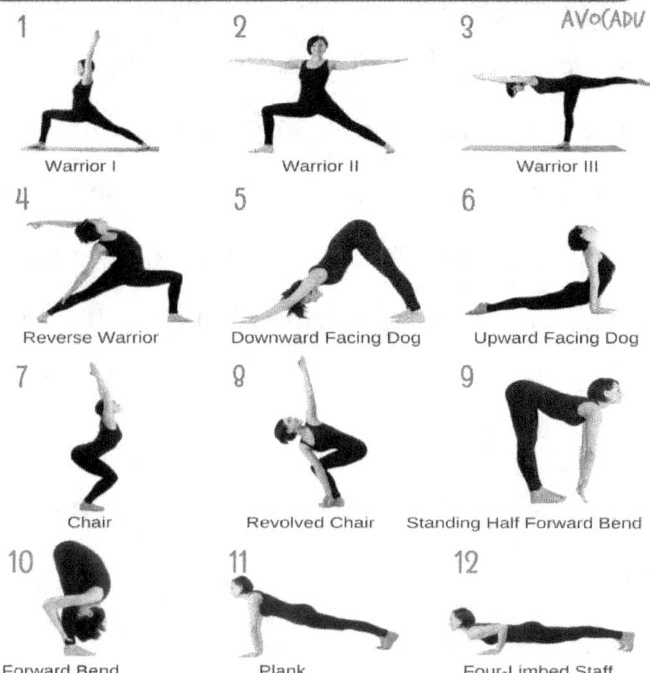

Conclusion: Empowering Change and Transformation

As we reach the culmination of this journey towards understanding obesity, health, and wellness, it becomes clear that empowering change and transformation is not only possible but essential for achieving lasting well-being.

Throughout this book, we have explored the multifaceted nature of obesity, its underlying causes, and the profound impact it has on individuals and society as a whole.

We have delved into the science behind obesity, dissecting its mechanisms, exploring its consequences, and uncovering the role of lifestyle factors in its prevention and management.

From understanding the hormonal mechanisms driving obesity to unravelling the complexities of dietary choices and lifestyle habits, we have equipped ourselves with knowledge and insights to embark on a transformative journey towards better health.

By embracing evidence-based strategies, adopting a holistic approach to wellness, and harnessing the power of lifestyle medicine and mind-body practices, we can pave the way for meaningful change and sustainable transformation.

It is essential to recognize that the path to health and wellness is not a one-size-fits-all approach. Each individual's journey is unique, shaped by personal experiences, genetic predispositions, and environmental factors.

However, by arming ourselves with knowledge, cultivating self-awareness, and making informed choices, we can take proactive steps towards achieving our health goals and living our best lives.

Empowering change and transformation requires a shift in mind-set a willingness to challenge ingrained habits, embrace new perspectives, and prioritize self-care.

It is a journey of self-discovery, resilience, and growth, where each step forward brings us closer to our vision of optimal health and well-being.

As we reflect on the insights gained from this exploration, let us remember that change is possible, and transformation is within reach.

By taking ownership of our health, making conscious choices, and supporting one another on this journey, we can create a ripple effect of positive change that extends far beyond ourselves.

In closing, let us embark on this journey of empowerment, armed with knowledge, fuelled by determination, and guided by the belief that we have the power to transform our health and our lives.

Together, let us embrace change, cultivate resilience, and embark on a path towards lasting well-being.

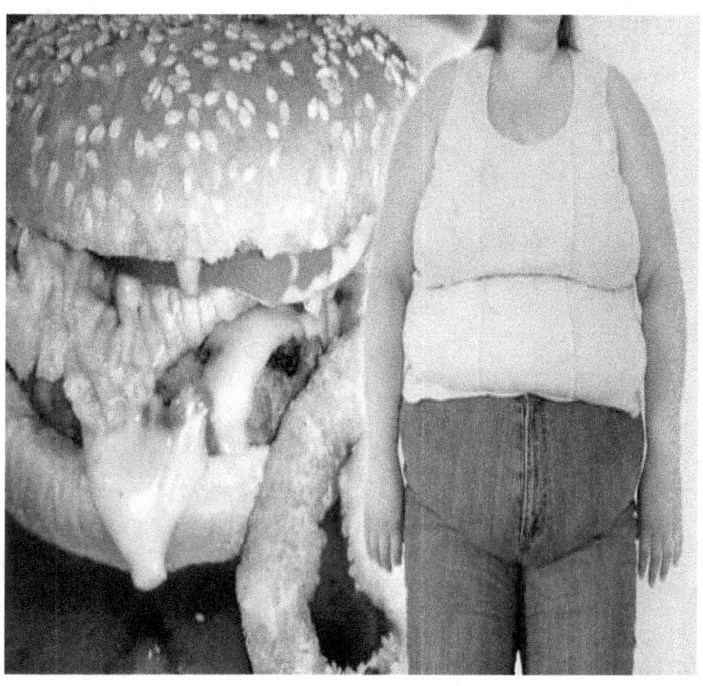